The Power of Intermittent Fasting

How to Lose Pounds the Simple and Easy Way

By: Gary Hatfield

9781680322347

PUBLISHERS NOTES

Disclaimer – Speedy Publishing LLC

This publication is intended to provide helpful and informative material. It is not intended to diagnose, treat, cure, or prevent any health problem or condition, nor is intended to replace the advice of a physician. No action should be taken solely on the contents of this book. Always consult your physician or qualified health-care professional on any matters regarding your health and before adopting any suggestions in this book or drawing inferences from it.

The author and publisher specifically disclaim all responsibility for any liability, loss or risk, personal or otherwise, which is incurred as a consequence, directly or indirectly, from the use or application of any contents of this book.

Any and all product names referenced within this book are the trademarks of their respective owners. None of these owners have sponsored, authorized, endorsed, or approved this book.

Always read all information provided by the manufacturers' product labels before using their products. The author and publisher are not responsible for claims made by manufacturers.

This book was originally printed before 2014. This is an adapted reprint by Speedy Publishing LLC with newly updated content designed to help readers with much more accurate and timely information and data.

Speedy Publishing LLC

40 E Main Street, Newark, Delaware, 19711

Contact Us: 1-888-248-4521

Website: http://www.speedypublishing.co

REPRINTED Paperback Edition: ISBN: 9781680322347

Manufactured in the United States of America

DEDICATION

I dedicate this book to my family. They are the source of my inspiration.

TABLE OF CONTENTS

Chapter 1- Is Intermittent Fasting Real?

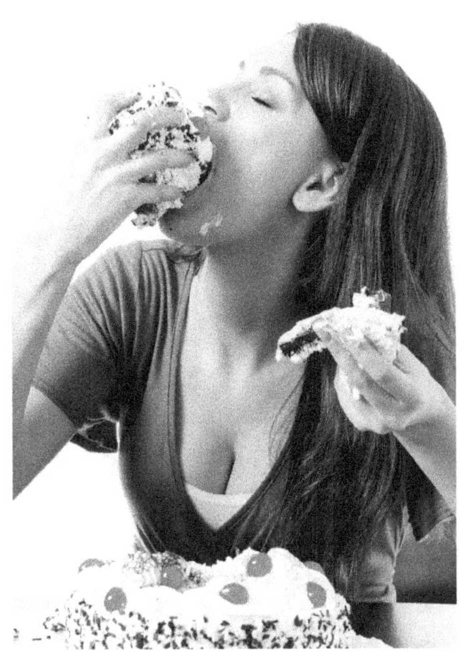

It's almost impossible to hide from the news and discussion about the obesity epidemic that's taking both lives and shattering the quality of life worldwide. It's in the papers, on television and being blogged about on the internet almost endlessly.

If that's not enough, unless you're blind it's hard to walk the streets of any big city or small town and not see the end product of this epidemic first hand.

The hard brutal truth is that people are getting fatter and fatter and this is a real health crisis that only a fool could ignore.

There are plenty of reasons for this here are just the most blindingly apparent...

Many People Eat Way too Much Way too Often.

It's a hard truth that can't be escaped. The human body wasn't designed by nature to eat as much and as often as most people do. This packs on the flabby pounds as our bodies, which are machines that were designed for survival in not so great circumstances are pampered and overfed in a cushy and soft environment. Remove a bit of hunger from our lives and we will pack on fat and pack it on at lightning speed.

A Widespread Avoidance of Exercise.

After overeating the next huge issue is under exercising. Having less physical jobs as well as social lives that revolve around the digital rather than the physical once again takes our bodies away from what they were designed for: running, lifting, hunting and playing. The less muscle we carry the lower our metabolism which means even more fat is packed on. Do you see a pattern developing?

Lack of Quality Sleep.

The first two obesity builders contribute to the third. Poor diet and lack of exercise offer the fast track to broken sleep patterns which have been shown in more studies than can be counted to also wreck metabolism and pack on fat. Sleepless nights tossing and turning quickly equal an ugly spare tire of flab around the waist.

Medicine and Drugs

Coming along with our increasingly over medicated society are the side effects of all these medications, which commonly include weight gain and lethargy. Cultures that approach health more naturally and holistically have largely avoided this issue and have been also able to avoid the obesity related health concerns that come along with it. Our societies for the most part haven't figured this out yet.

These are just some of the many reasons the obesity plague is spreading in such a quick and deadly manner. There's plenty more, trust me.

The question stands - what can we do about it? How can we turn the tide against obesity?

The answer is, of course, diet and exercise. There are plenty of diverse ideas about both, some good and a few bad.

This guide offers what I feel may be the perfect solution to a vast majority of people's struggle with putting on fat. It's fairly simple and packed with power, in line with both nature and common sense. Most importantly it works and works almost like magic.

It's called the Feast and Famine Diet and it can change your life for the better. After reading this you will be armed with all you need to know about Feast and Famine to make it work and get the lean and healthy body of your dreams.

Get ready this is going to be a blast!

The Feast and Famine Diet may be new in name, but in practice has been with us for quite some time. It's the latest tweak on an area of diet programs and ideas less catchingly referred to as Intermittent Fasting.

Intermittent Fasting is the rage in health, fitness and weight loss circles with its ideas making it to publication and wide practice. It's popular because it works!

The Power of Intermittent Fasting

Here's the important guiding principle of Feast and Famine, what gives the diet its power. Try not to stray too far from this foundation if you expect to reap the full rewards of Feast and Famine...

Choose Your Fasting Schedule

There are two approaches generally. The first is alternating Feast days with Famine days, which is personally the method I have seen produce the best weight loss results. The second variant and this is what you will see in intermittent fasting diets like the 5:2 Diets is to eat normally five days and fast two. Our Guide's information works well with both methods, although once again I prefer the first for best long term results as well as ease of use and likelihood of being able to stick with Feast and Famine.

Feasting Guidelines

There's not many. I suggest broadly not eating anything that's junk food or packed with empty calories especially if you are looking to burn off a lot of weight. This will also safeguard your overall health, which is important isn't it? Make sure you get in your fruit and vegetables, but don't be afraid to indulge without binge eating. The fact you have more food freedom at least half the time will make your Famine days much easier to manage psychology.

And succeeding on any diet, Feast and Famine included, is 90% a mental game. In this mental dieting game no diet stacks the deck more in your favor than Feast and Famine.

Famine Guidelines

For those needing to drop serious pounds, 500 calories a day on Famine days is a good starting point. This can be adjusted as needed once your weight loss goals are met. Most Feast and Famine enthusiasts like to stay around this area to continue to both reap the health benefits of fasting and to also be able to maintain their Feasting freedom on their Feast days.

* Stay Hydrated. Fasting expert or if you have never fasted in any form before alike, I cannot stress enough the importance of staying hydrated. When your body detoxes on your Famine days and starts to move out some of the junk you have built up, it will go much smoother if you are drinking a proper amount of water. Ignore this advice and you may just experience some stomach pains, along with the lethargy and weakness that always comes with dehydration regardless of your diet plan.

One of the greatest strengths of intermittent fasting and the Feast and Famine Diet is its simplicity. No diet logs, carbohydrate manipulation schemes and other complications. It works much more dramatically than diets that you need flow charts to follow too. If you can't stick to Feast and Famine it has nothing to do with being confused, but with a lack of will power, self discipline and most of all desire. I think you have those covered, don't you?

Every good idea got its start somewhere. The every other day Feast and Famine Diet has had its way paved for it by earlier intermittent fasting protocols, some a big influence and others not so much, but who still deserve credit for being forward thinkers.

Let's take a look at the history of diets that have come before Feast and Famine and see what we can learn from them. Knowledge is power after all. We have already seen in the mirror and felt in our bodies - that Feast and Famine works big time, we have these pace setters to thank for their experiments and innovations!

First the Warrior.

Make no mistake; Ori Hofmekler is certainly a unique guy. Artist, writer and ex-special forces soldier who ran a short lived fitness magazine that was published by a famous Men's magazine company.

During his time as editor in chief he was exposed to the often conflicting ideas of a who's who of dieting gurus of the time, which landed him an obsession with getting to the truth about fat loss.

A few years later came the Warrior Diet book which promotes a 16 hour daily fast followed by a 8 hour eating period. Overall consensus was that it worked, but most people feel the Warrior Diet is difficult to maintain, much more so than every other day fasting ala Feast and Famine. Either way Ori definitely gets credit for the modern birth of intermittent fasting and has served as a great influence on most everyone's ideas who are working with these methods.

Eat Stop Eat.

Eat Stop Eat has been an intermittent fasting dieting method promoted most recently by Brad Pillon. Brad pushes the idea of one or two, zero calorie days a week, the rest of the days eating normally. Once again it's effective and close to what we suggest, but our experience has shown going down to 500 calories every other day is much more effective and manageable than a few days of no calories at all. Not many seem to be able to stick with Eat Stop Eat for long in our experience.

The 5:2 Diet.

This is the diet plan most closely related to Feast and Famine and also closest to us on the time line. It's wildly popular in Europe and is gaining ground in places like Hollywood in the USA.

Five days of normal eating followed by two days of reduced calories. Very powerful and all our ideas here work well with the 5:2 Diet. Our opinion holds every other day Feast and Famine is a better fat burner without added psychological tolls. Follow this Guide's advice and I think you will agree!

That's the recent history of intermittent fasting leading us to where we are today. Feast and Famine is the present and I have no doubt it will proudly stand the test of time. It torches fat, is easy to follow, requires really no added expenses in its purest form and promotes over all vibrant health. What's there not to love about Feast and Famine? It's perfect for the health enthusiast who wants to get lean and look great.

Chapter 2- Intermittent Fasting: Feast and Famine Diet

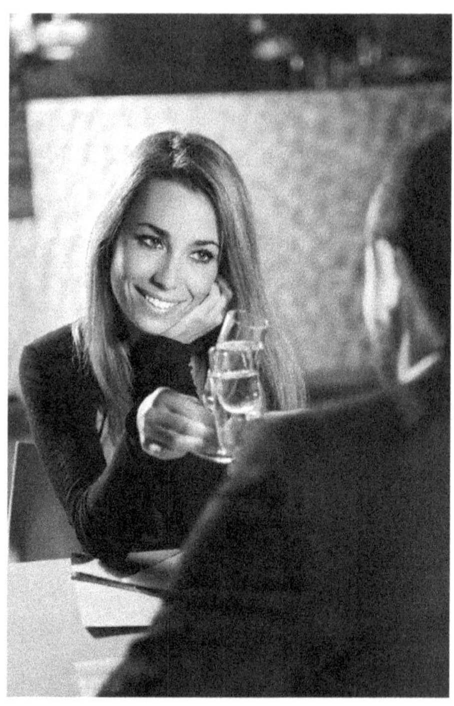

Any diet requires a bit of preparation at first, Feast and Famine is certainly not an exception. I will say it requires much less preparation by the nature of Feast and Famine than any other diet I can think of and you won't have to jump many hurdles, do any real expensive shopping or experience any of the other more traditional diet headaches.

Here are some tips to get yourself ready to get the most out our plan...

Read and Understand This Guide

It's pretty short so why not even read it twice. I've done my best to keep it fluff free and all the information and tips will make your journey at intermittent fasting Feast and Famine style much, much easier. If you like to read check out some of the books in our history chapter and you may find some other ideas you'd like to incorporate after you've done straight Feast and Famine for a bit.

If Possible At First Food Shop More Often

Here's a trick I used in the beginning days of my intermittent fasting experiments and I've suggested to many of my friends and clients who have given it high praise too. Only keep enough food on hand for the days needs.

On Feasting days you will have the pleasure of picking out some new treat to indulge in and on Famine days you won't be as tempted to cheat than you would be if the refrigerator is packed with snacks.

Now if you live rurally, or have a large family this may be less practical, but if you can do it I guarantee it will give you a big advantage over those who ignore this tip.

If You Skip A Day Just Get Right Back On Schedule

This diet is about freedom and abundance not restriction. If you have a family event, a date or even a slight slip up on a Famine day just get right back in action the next day and reduce your calories. No master dietary equations are fouled or other nonsense.

Now don't make a habit of this or you may end up seeing less than optimal results, but once in a while is perfectly fine. This automatic leeway is built into the Feast and Famine program making it not a diet you can "fail" at if you stumble while getting into the groove, or any other time really!

Throw Out Your Past Diet Experiences

Feast and Famine requires a whole new view of dieting, so in all likelihood your past dieting experiences positive and especially negative don't offer a whole lot of relevance. I'd suggest you file them away and don't let them influence what you are doing here and now. This attitude, not only in dieting and fitness, but also in other areas of life can break chains and open up doors. See what you think.

Are you feeling more ready to begin? You should be because there's a bright, fit and happy new you waiting at the end of the Feast and Famine road. And it's a road not particularly long in most cases or even exceedingly difficult. You've taken the first step by reading this Guide, don't turn back now!

Benefits of Intermittent Fasting

The Feast and Famine Diet brings a load of benefits some more obvious than others. Are you ready to take a look? I think you'll find them really exciting. If radically reducing fat while also basking in these health benefits doesn't interest someone looking to transform their body for the better I'm not sure what will!

Quickly Cut Body Fat Safely

This is why most people will explore the Feast and Famine approach to diet. You can expect to see the fat melt off as long as you take your Famine days seriously. Eat too much on those days and you are obviously missing the point. We know this works, we've seen it and now even better news - science backs it up!

Recent University of Illinois research has shown in those following alternate day reduced calorie plans (inline with our Guide's recommendations) lost significantly more fat than those eating normally and following the same exercise protocols. It's a plus to be on the right side of science when, sadly, they most often trail far behind the true health and diet vanguard!

Easy To Follow And Manage

The next ground breaking benefit of Feast and Famine is how easy it is to follow and manage. I've touched on this already, but it truly bears repeating. Anyone who has counted carbs on a ketogenic diet like Atkins or the many others I'm sure will quickly agree! Once you figure out in your head what your 500 or 600 calories on famine days looks like you are set. No calculators or complications, period.

Enhanced Mental Function

Yes, we suspected it, but science has backed us up again. Reduced weekly calories (which is what you get with the Feast and Famine Diet) leads to increased focus, better memory and other enhanced cognitive function according to Mark Mattson's research for the Lancet. These effects may even carry over into the fight against Alzheimer's disease and other similar huge health concerns which Mattson is exploring further.

Improve Insulin Levels

One of the reasons why many people pack on and find it so hard to lose body fat is their out of whack insulin levels. The Feast and Famine approach optimizes insulin levels for healthy fat loss, which just adds to the amount of fat already being cut from the calorie reduction and heightened metabolism we've already touched on.

One of the surprise benefits of this approach is the new found time you find available on Famine days. Small meals and no constant snacking or grazing frees up a shocking amount of time and energy that can be used positively elsewhere. I've found, and others have confirmed this, that some of our most creative and productive days turn out again and again to be famine days! Far from not having energy you end up filled with it!

The Feast and Famine Diet approach is packed with benefits, physical, mental and even social. It's hard to even think of anything, but a small drawback or two and then only for those who are lacking in the desire to "get lean" department. This is truly a method that changes lives for the best.

CHAPTER 3- WHAT YOU SHOULD AVOID IN INTERMITTENT FASTING

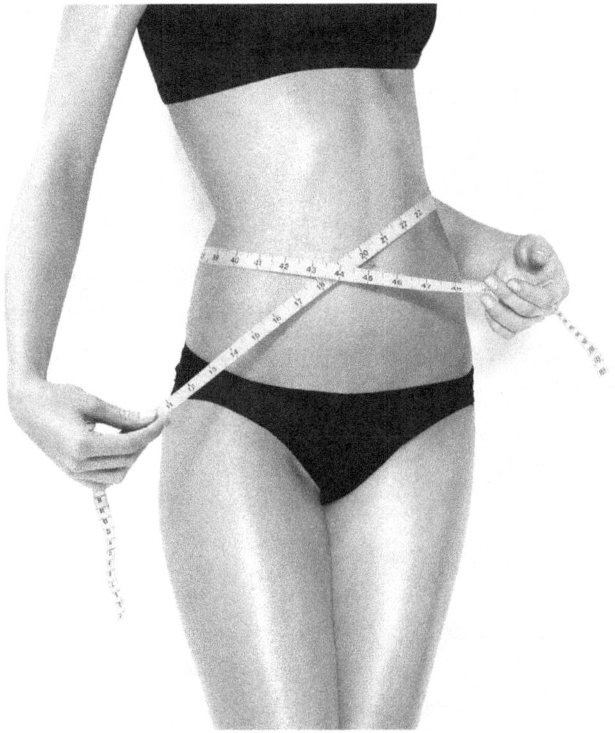

Now just because the Feast and Famine Diet is easy to understand and simple to apply to your lifestyle doesn't mean it's easy for all to practice or it's impossible to make mistakes. In fact some mistakes with intermittent fasting are fairly common among beginners, let's go over them and see if you can't avoid these pitfalls before you make them rather than after. A few of these I even learned the hard way!

Pigging Out on Too Much on Junk Food

Let's be serious for a second on the subject of getting lean and healthy. While we are allowed and encouraged to eat loosely and enjoyably on Feast days this doesn't mean we have a license to eat completely like a glutton. So if you are not losing weight the way you'd like to be and are eating endless chips, ice cream and candy on your Feast days tighten up your diet and eat healthier.

You should be striving to optimize your health anyway shouldn't you?

Being Scared to Death of Hunger

No one has ever starved to death eating 500 calories or less every other day. Nor have they damaged their body in any way. So if you are experiencing great stress and discomfort over being hungry every other day, it's time to gain more control over your mind. This is done by developing your will power doing things like following this diet even when you would rather not be, focusing on your desired end result. Be tough and be rewarded.

Eating Too Much On Famine Days

Let's not play games, 500 calories or less means 500 calories or less. If you are eating clean on your Feast days and still not losing weight it likely means you are eating too much on Famine days. Cut down what you are eating and if you must check the calorie counts to make sure you are at 500 calories or under.

Reducing Your Level of Activity

It's tempting for some to slow down their activities on Famine days. Don't fall into this. In fact with a little Feast and Famine experience under your belt you will realize Famine days actually free up more energy and you should strive to be even more active. Doing more is almost always better than doing nothing as long as you can do it safely.

Putting Yourself Unnecessarily Around People Who Don't Respect Your Diet Efforts.

Apart from close friends and family who it would be difficult to avoid, it's a downer to be around people who try to talk negatively about or discourage you from meeting your Feast and Famine goals. Again dieting is 90% mental so don't let other people mess with your mental game. It's annoying, defeatist and unnecessary!

These common beginner mistakes are all easy to avoid and if you stumble it's ok just keep going. The Feast and Famine Diet has been designed to be both effective, open and user friendly. A little bit of self-reflection and you are quickly back on course and seizing the body and life of your dreams!

Chapter 4- Eat More To Lose Weight Principle

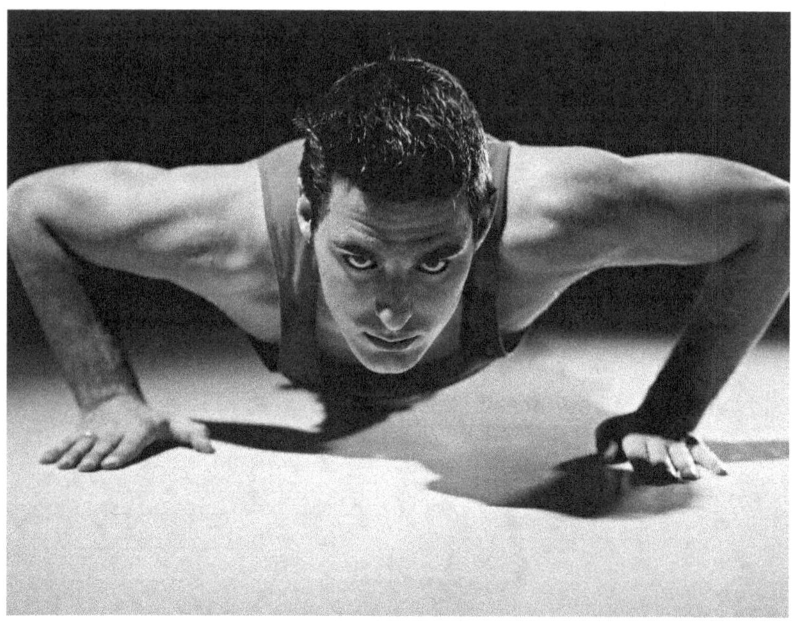

The Feast and Famine Feast Day! Now comes the fun part, my friends! Let's dig deep into a sample Feast day while we are following the Feast and Famine Diet.

This is taken from my own lifestyle and from a period of time when I was consistently losing weight as fast as I ever had every week without fail. My metabolism has never been superhuman either, so rest assured if this has worked for me it's very, very likely to work for you as well (with portion sizes adjusted if you are female, of course.)

Read on and enjoy. I hope it gets you filled with enthusiasm! You will notice I'm not including calories, because who counts calories on a Feast day?! I sure don't and you shouldn't either.

Breakfast

Breakfast is regarded by many nutrition experts as being the most important meal of the day. It's also a meal I've neglected most of my life due to the perils of enjoying sleeping in. Intermittent fasting has cleared that up - after a 500 calorie day I can't wait to really eat a substantial breakfast! I must say I feel much more ready for action after a full force breakfast.

4 Eggs Scrambled. I choose to go with whole eggs for hormonal optimization's sake, but often mix up the ways the eggs are prepared.

Fresh Tomato, Onion and Jalapeno Salsa. Extra hot and used as a condiment on top of my eggs.

4 pieces of Turkey Bacon. I will eat other styles of bacon when turkey bacon isn't available.

4oz of Steak Sauteed in Frying Pan. I only add this when I really want to indulge or if I feel like I need the extra protein for muscle building purposes.

8oz Milk. Whole milk is also great for guys looking to naturally boost their hormonal advantage,

Snack

A few hand fulls of Organic Almonds

Small Spinach Salad. I don't use dressing beyond olive oil and garlic and sometimes toss in some tomatoes, onion and cucumber depending what's on hand.

Lunch

Medium Baked Potato. I dress the potato with a bit of butter and garlic.

Two 6oz Grilled Chicken Breasts. Sometimes plain or sometimes with salsa on top if I have extra from breakfast.

Small Side of Mixed Vegetables. Snack

More Almonds!

Dinner

10oz Grilled Lean Steak. Plain beyond salt and pepper.

Small side salad or spinach salad. Side Portion of White or Brown Rice.

As much Green Tea as I'd like to drink sweetened with pure stevia.

Occasionally a desert of organic sorbet, a small addiction of mine!

Snack

My after dinner snack is pretty wide open within reason. If I eat chips I make sure to not go overboard.

Vanilla Whey Protein shake made with half whole milk and half almond milk. I drink this right before bed.

This is just a sample Feast and Famine Feast day, but it should give you a great idea of what's possible when we eat smartly and abundantly. The real eye opener is when you eat like this half the time and still see the fat melting away. That's when you will become a full force Feast and Famine true believer!

Famine Day

Now after seeing a sample Feast and Famine Feast day it's time for a sample of the flip side - the all important Famine day where we will fast eating vastly reduced calories activating our metabolism, our "skinny gene" and setting ourselves up for both body transformation and all the other health benefits we have already discussed. This is again, from my own personal experience and the daily calorie total is focused on the magic number of 500 calories. I think you will find this a very manageable day that will hardly leave you suffering.

Pre-Breakfast

16oz Spring Water immediately upon wakening.

A cup of Fresh Coffee, no milk or cream sweetened with stevia. 0 calories.

Breakfast

A second cup of Fresh Coffee, no milk or cream sweetened with stevia. 0 calories.

8oz Spring Water.

Now this doesn't seem like much of a breakfast, but I prefer to sleep in a bit and save my calories for lunch and dinner. This is my own personal choice and you may choose to distribute your calories differently if you are more of a morning person!

Snack

8oz Green Tea sweetened with stevia. 0 calories.

12oz Spring water. Lunch

Finally time to get in some food, paying special intention

NOT to overdo it. This is the meal when many feel most tempted, since while eating a small dinner you know a large breakfast is coming up relatively quickly. Don't give in!

Two medium hard boiled eggs. Once again I like to make sure I eat whole eggs every day to maximize my hormonal optimization plan. You have the option of egg whites, egg beaters and so on. 175 Calories.

Two slices Whole Wheat Toast. Sometimes I eat the eggs on the toast and sometimes as a side depending on mood. 115 Calories.

A cup of Fresh Coffee, no milk or cream sweetened with stevia. 0 calories.

8oz spring water.

Total Lunch calories: 290 give or take.

Snack

8oz Green Tea sweetened with stevia. 0 calories. Yes, I do love caffeine on Famine day in case you were wondering. It serves to boost energy, raise metabolism and even acts as a mild appetite suppressant.

12oz Spring water. Dinner

Half a cup (after cooked) Spaghetti with a small amount of low fat / low calorie butter, salt, pepper and garlic. 150 calories.

One slice whole wheat toast. 55 calories.

12oz Spring Water.

Total calorie intake for the day roughly 495 calories. This puts right where we are hoping to be on a Famine day. I repeat these meals often since they are pretty much decision free and simple to prepare. They can also easily be ordered in all but the most incompetent of restaurants!

One last bit of advice - take a half hour on Sunday and figure out your five hundred calorie and below meals for the week rather than just trying to wing it and guess how many calories you are eating on Famine days on the fly.

This will end up equating in much more weight loss over the long term and also save you a few headaches and a bit of possible confusion too. When in doubt repeat meals! Don't worry about getting bore a Feast day is less than 24 hours away!

Chapter 5- The Proper Food for your Intermittent Fasting Diet

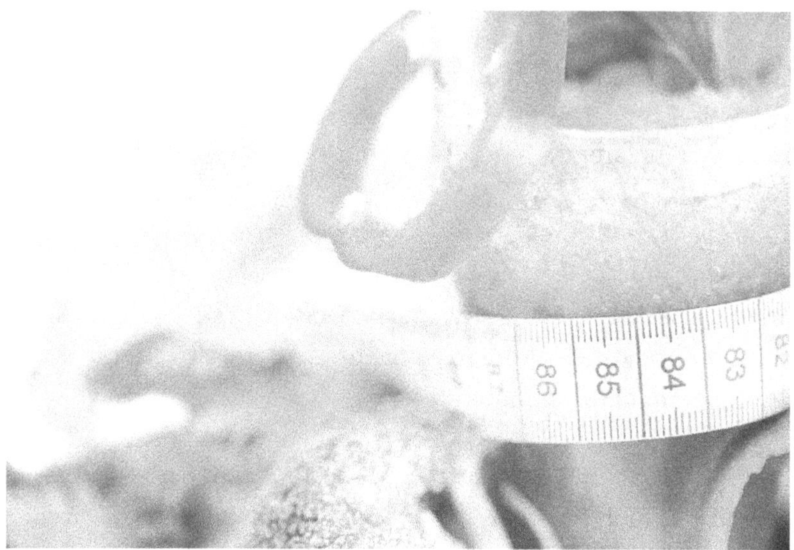

Now that we hopefully have agreed that the Feast and Famine Diet is more than do-able after looking at a sample Feast day and a sample Famine day I thought I'd share with you a few more intermittent fasting insider's secrets.

The fine art of shopping while following Feast and Famine. Although all of us develop our style of eating while on the diet which best suits our individual needs I've found having an experience veteran's shopping list can provide some helpful guidelines. So are you ready to go shopping Feast and Famine style? Let's do it!

Here's what we are packing our shopping cart with...

Non-hormonal Chicken Breasts. I'm a bit of a chicken addict and don't think I could live without it. I eat chicken at least once a day on Feast days, sometimes twice. I think of chicken as a sort of "neutral" protein that can be prepared in so many ways it's wise to fall in love with.

Make sure the fat is trimmed off!

Non-hormonal Grass Fed Lean Beef. Another Feast day favorite, especially when I'm hitting it more heavily in the gym. When you are looking to put on muscle while cutting fat on Feast and Famine aim for around 1 gram of protein for every pound you weigh.

Eggs. As you've seen eggs are on the meal agenda often for both Feast and Famine days. Don't skip them, unless you are one of the few who can't stomach the thought of them!

A variety of Pasta. Organic Spinach

Organic Leaf Lettuce. I should add organic produce is not a must, but I try to stick with it when I can.

Tomatoes.

Onions.

Miso soup. Miso soup is great for a change of pace on Famine days and has been shown in research to have all sorts of regenerative and health boosting qualities. Plus it tastes great too!

Green Tea. Essential. Green Tea is great for an extra fat burning boost, is inexpensive and calorie free.

Coffee. Spring Water.

Whey Protein. I've tried to avoid any supplement recommendations as the Feast and Famine Diet works great without them, but a good protein shake is the one exception. Keep your protein levels high and you will have no worries at all about losing muscle while cutting body fat.

Stevia. A all natural and calorie free sweetener which will make you forget sugar ever even existed. A true gift from above.

Almonds. A go to snack.

Now a look at this list reveals that avoiding overly processed and junk food isn't a bad idea and you can still really Feast without it. That way if you go a bit crazy at a friend's or eating out occasionally your body won't even notice it.

Buying too many terrible food choices probably sends the wrong message to your subconscious and may set up many for binge eating and failure. Some intermittent fasting experts disagree, but this is what my own personal experience has revealed. After you move beyond the beginner stage feel free to experiment!

CHAPTER 6- INTERMITTENT FASTING & YOUR LIFESTYLE

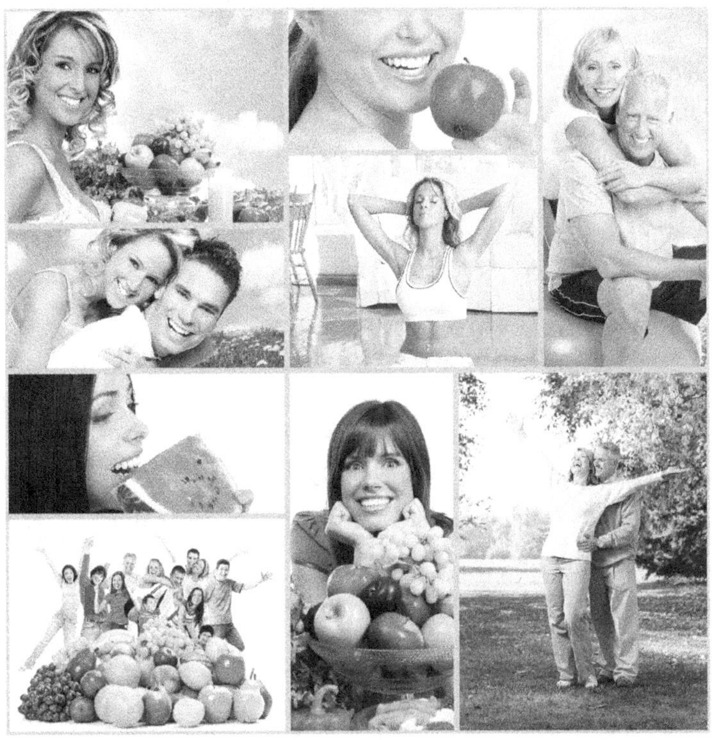

The only way to really lose weight and keep it off is to make the mental switch from thinking in terms of short term dieting to the more dynamic perspective of making lasting healthy lifestyle choices.

Feast and Famine is the perfect tool to help you make that change. In fact after studying and experimenting with every major diet of the last decade, I can honestly say none in my opinion are better suited for a long term lifestyle choice than intermittent fasting and Feast and Famine. It's easy to manage, inexpensive to follow, relatively pleasant and enjoyable and very, very powerful. This covers nearly every category of a dream long term eating plan check list I can think of!

Here's some tips in incorporating Feast and Famine into your lifestyle long term...

Celebrate Your Successes With Feast And Famine.

Thinking positive and choosing to focus on the positive changes you have made while intermittent fasting will go a long way in solidifying it as a part of your lasting lifestyle. Try your best to not dwell on any poor weeks or bumps in the road you may experience. This will pay off huge dividends both in weight loss and in life. Again 90% of the game is mental, let's not forget.

Recruit Those Closest To You To Lend A Hand

Making your significant other close friends and family aware of how Feast and Famine works and letting them know you could use their help encouraging you to be disciplined on Famine days will help this healthy lifestyle really cement itself in place. Some may even choose to take up the Feast and Famine flag themselves when they see how great you look and feel. That's when you know you are really onto something!

Take Off A Week Off Every Few Months

Everyone needs a vacation occasionally. This will prevent burn out and give yourself a great pat on the back after months of discipline. If you can time your vacation from Feast and Famine with a real vacation from work or school even better! I've found a week off really helps recharge enthusiasm's batteries and allows me to plunge back into the Feast and Famine lifestyle full force.

Keep Expanding Your Knowledge Of Intermittent Fasting

A final way to make sure you stick with Feast and Famine as a lifestyle choice is to keep your brain engaged in learning new knowledge about intermittent fasting in all its forms. Join some forums, follow the news and the blogs and if you go to a gym make friends with others living this way of life. This will continually confirm what you are doing is both healthy and a good choice. It's always a good idea to have as big a support circle as possible.

Even if you take up Feast and Famine to lose some weight quickly planning to go back to your old ways of eating, let me warn you, you may very well end up hooked and sticking around for the duration. The good news is your body will be much healthier and look much better for your efforts. Breaking from the norm into a lifestyle that gets the most out of body and mind is a benefit that's priceless. Embrace it!

Your Journey

Thanks for taking the time to read our Guide and I truly hope you have found it helpful and eye opening. I have no doubt if you throw your focus into the Feast and Famine Diet you will achieve your weight loss goals and much more.

That said when do you plan to start? If you just hesitated you may be experiencing the greatest foe of achieving the body of your dreams of them all - the evil called procrastination. Before I leave let me share with you some tips that can help you slay that beast and begin your own transformation story today!

The Feast and Famine Diet requires no special food, no supplements and no information, really, beyond this Guide to work and work well. So what are you waiting for? Start Feast and Famine right NOW. The only thing stopping you is your own inertia. Banish any thoughts of tomorrow or next week. Once again make a decision and start NOW.

Expose Your Excuses

Do you have reoccurring excuses why you can't start intermittent fasting today? Say these excuses out loud so you can hear how ridiculously self defeating they are. If you are still in doubt write them down and burn them as you free yourself from limiting beliefs.

Look At Yourself Naked In The Mirror.

If you are fat the mirror and a lack of clothes won't lie. Remind yourself your body won't change into something more pleasing until you first make a decision to change it and then second move forward with action in support of that decision.

That action is to wisely adopt the Feast and Famine Diet. If not you will likely look the same, if not worse, than you did in the mirror in the days, weeks, months and years to come. This may sound harsh, but a harsh truth is much better than a pleasant falsehood.

Quit Time Wasters.

Do you need so much social media, television or playing video games when your body isn't where you desire it to be? Are you putting the easy and distracting before the vital and important? If so why? Break the trance, quit the time wasters and build the new you NOW!

Write Your Goals Down As Clearly And Detailed As Possible.

There's a certain magic about the written word, especially when it comes to setting and achieving goals. This magic is even more pronounced when the written words are your own. Write down your goals big and small, read them and embrace Feast and Famine as a means to carry you in the direction you need to be headed. There isn't a success coach or sports psychologist alive who would argue against that advice! You shouldn't either.

Are you psyched about moving forward with Feast and Famine? I knew you would be. This could be a day you look back on decades from now and say "that's where I committed to serious life enhancing change!" The things offered by this lifestyle are just that serious.

CHAPTER 7- EATING OVERLOAD WITH THE RIGHT FOOD

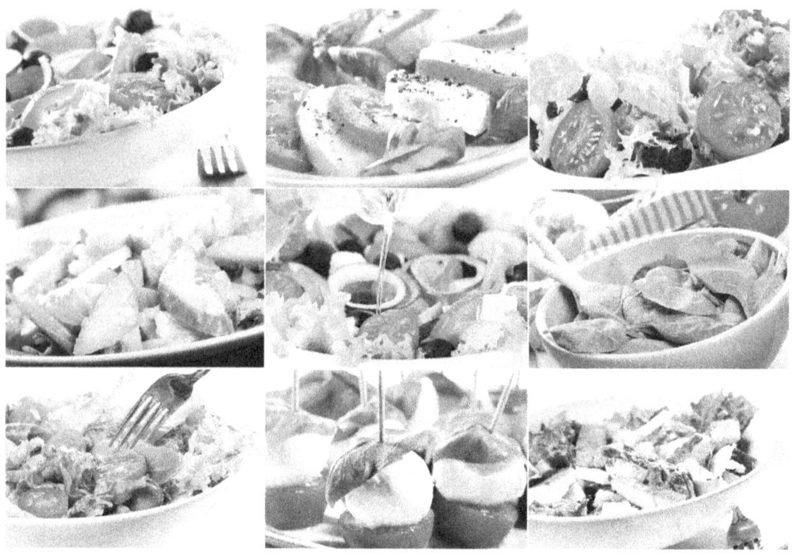

There are no such things as miracle treatments for a weight loss problem. Of course, it is possible to become slim through the use of fad diets, but you will not be healthy because crash diets deny you nutrients that are necessary for your body to function properly.

It weakens your health and what's more you are likely to go back to your former eating habits since the fad diet taught you nothing. You will be having the same problem again and again. Worse, according to studies people who have undergone repetitive weight loss diets, then became permanently overweight, and are in worse health than those who hadn't tried solving their weight problems at all.

Change Your Lifestyle

Changing your lifestyle is actually the most effective way of losing weight and staying healthy. A switch from a calorie-loaded diet to a low calorie diet is a must. You do not actually have to reduce food intake, just eat healthful foods - more vegetables and fruits, lean meats, whole grains and others.

Regular exercise should also help you lose weight as well as maintaining good health. Since you are taking in fewer calories from your diet, your workouts should be burning fat deposits in your body.

The workouts may not be even programmed. Sports and games like tennis or basketball are excellent exercise and if you feel like other forms of exercise are a chore. You can actually enjoy the games though, especially when you play with friends, which means turning exercise into a habit will not be difficult.

The process of getting you down to your appropriate weight through the natural method may be slow, but you feel good the whole time and maintaining gains does not require doing anything outside of your established daily routine.

One Step at a Time

In a world where fast food is considered a real meal, no wonder there are so many people in a bad shape. The rate of obese people is a cause for alarm but this can all change if everyone gets educated on healthy eating habits.

The secret to healthy eating is all about balance. It's having all the right nutrients, vitamins and calories in one meal. There's really no need to deprive yourself from food that you like. It's about having all of these foods, but in moderation. Like the old saying goes, Too much of anything is bad. This can be applied greatly to the food you eat.

The truth is, what you consume everyday greatly affects your whole attitude and energy level for the whole day. Sure it is convenient but there's so much more to life than a cheeseburger meal or Chinese food take out. It's tasty and you can't help craving it, but experimenting in your kitchen can easily result in the best meal of your life.

So here are some tips for healthy eating habits for a better you:

If you are just starting to change into a healthier lifestyle, then do it slowly. Your body has been accustomed to old ways and if you change drastically, it is likely that you will also give up easily.

Eat At Home

Whenever you eat out, you do not have any control on the portions that you will have. You might end up eating more than you need to.

Stop Counting the Calories

Do not be obsessed about that. Instead, look at food in terms of color and freshness. Greens are always good. Colorful fruits are also great for a person's body. These are the food that your body needs more of. So do not feel afraid to eat more of these.

Do Not Skip Meals

If your goal is to lose weight, then it is much better to eat small portions of food 5- 6 times a day. Skipping meals will only retain the fat in your body and may result in overeating.

Snack Healthy

When you're feeling hungry, instead of reaching out for the cupcake, grab that carrot stick instead. Some good examples of food to snack on are fruits, nuts, raisins, cranberries, whole grain crackers, etc.

Enjoy Your Meal

Do not rush the eating process. Take your time and chew your food slowly. When you're already feeling full, then stop eating. Listen to what your body tells you.

Remember To Drink a Lot of Water

Sometimes people confuse thirst with hunger and eat when all they needed was just a glass of water. Drinking water is also good for cleansing the body from toxins and helps in having better digestion.

Along with these tips, you should always remember to have not just good eating habits but also a healthy lifestyle. This means making an effort to exercise regularly. If you are a smoker, then consider quitting and lastly, drink alcoholic beverages moderately.

Small Portions Several Times throughout the Day

Most experts say that there are many more benefits when it comes to losing weight if you eat 5-6 meals per day compared to 3 meals. Granted the meals are small, of course. The reason for this is because your body will have balanced levels of sugar in the blood. Meaning, you won't be feeling intense hunger. When a person is hungry, they tend to eat more than usual.

Eating smaller portions throughout the day will also reduce cholesterol. In studies done by experts, it was proven that having smaller meals consumed 6 times a day decreased cholesterol levels by 5 percent.

Fill that Plate Up With the Right Kind of Stuff

What a person eats greatly affects their weight loss or weight gain. This is why dietitians encourage people to go for quality over quantity.

 A good example is you might have eaten only crackers for lunch today but also had a huge jug of sweetened drinks. Then that sweetened drink is the culprit when it comes to your weight gain.

If you had a large bowl of fresh salad and water, then that would have been considered a better meal on a diet than the crackers with a sweetened drink.

It is much better for the body to take foods that are less in carbohydrates. Taking away bread, pasta, rice or potatoes and replacing it with vegetables will definitely help cut back on fat.

If you are the type of person who will feel full only if you see large portions of food on your plate, then the solution is to fill your plate with the right kind of food.

Think colorful fruits and vegetables. Deep colors means higher content of vitamins, minerals and antioxidants. All of these is what your body needs every day.

To commit to a long-term diet, it is important to like what you eat. If you hate the thought of just eating vegetables or fruits all day, then do some research on diet recipes. Eating meat is encouraged, so don't cut back on that. As long as it is not always deep fried, then it's still good.

It's really important to enjoy the process. Otherwise, you will easily go back to your old routine. Just remember, too much of anything is bad. Keep everything well balanced and eat only when your body is telling you it's hungry.

Chapter 8- Well-Planned Meal and Lose Weight Naturally

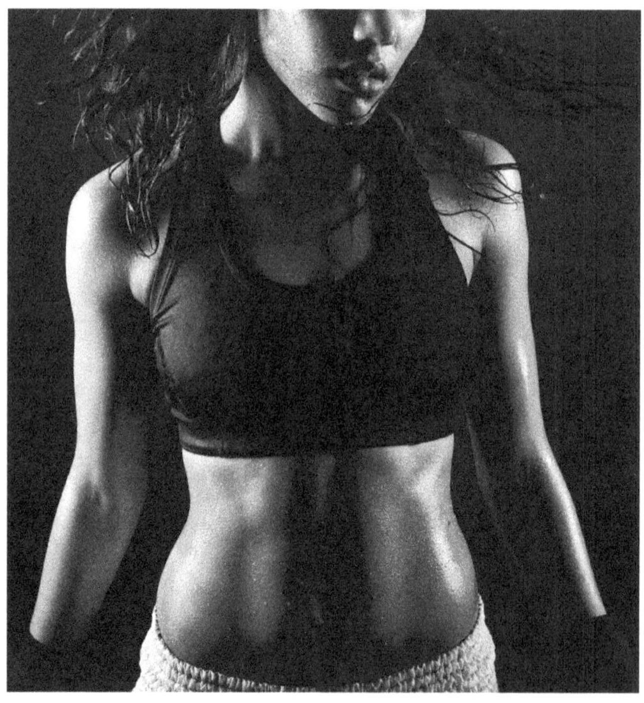

If you have noticed, just a quick search of weight loss on the Internet will immediately provide you with weight loss products like diet pills, weight loss programs and even gym memberships. These can cost a great deal of money and most of them are not even effective. So why not go back to basics and do the easiest and the cheapest thing you can do to lose weight: adopt a balanced diet.

Achieving a balanced diet includes eating the right kind and amount of food that will give you enough nutrients to sustain weight loss. Ideally, your diet should be heavier in fruits and vegetables, whole carbohydrates and low in dietary fats.

Additionally, lean proteins, and lots of water for hydration and exercise are important. Even though we all have different nutrient needs and metabolisms, all these factors are still important to achieve weight loss in the safest and cheapest way.

The Benefits of a Balanced Diet

Opting for a balanced diet to maintain a healthy weight is important in order to achieve weight loss since you are still supplying your body the right amount of vitamins and minerals it needs to function properly. When combined with consistent exercise, it is inevitable that you will lose weight without risking any health problems.

Maintaining a balanced diet with the aim of losing weight is beneficial as compared to products that promise a quick and easy way to weight loss. First, it lessens the risk of your developing cardiovascular diseases like heart diseases and diabetes. It can also aid you in controlling these conditions if ever you are suffering from one. This healthy regimen also promotes regular metabolism and a healthy digestive system, which will enable you to lose bad fats and absorb the good ones.

Aside from that, the choice of eating a balanced diet will definitely boost your confidence knowing that you will achieve your desired weight in the healthiest way possible.

How to Start Right

Starting out can be quite a challenge but it should be easy. Always remember the basics of eating more whole-carbohydrates by avoiding foods like chocolates, ice creams, chips, sodas, cookies, cakes and many others. These types of foods contain high amounts of sugar, cholesterol, salt and other unwanted substances.

These foods are also called 'empty calories' since they do not provide nutrients other than calories. Choose to drink fresh fruit juice instead of sodas, as they add approximately 500 calories more to your diet.

With that in mind, plan your meal correctly by adding more of the good kinds of food. You can have a high-fiber cereal with low-fat milk at breakfast, and then lunch would be a grilled turkey sandwich over whole wheat bread and a vegetable salad. Dinner can be baked fish and vegetables.

These are just a few of the simple dishes you can make and they are even easier to prepare. Just keep in mind that every meal should contain a variety of foods, such as fruits, lean proteins, vegetables and high-fiber carbohydrates.

The Science

Weight loss can sometimes be tiring. After thousands of dollars spent on diet programs with all efforts to cut-down calories, it seems that you are not losing weight as you expect it.

Of course, you will then have to check with your doctor or nutritionist to see why you are not losing that much weight and you will end up with 'the look' that strikes the paranoia out of you.

These are just few of the challenges you may encounter when you are into weight loss programs. It can get the best out of you depending on how you take all the challenges up. Well, there is a better way to actually achieve weight loss with 3 easy reminders.

1. There Is Such A Thing Called 'Real Carbohydrates'

The first thing you need to do is to identify your carbohydrate intake. All of us know that carbohydrates are the main source of energy as carbs are readily converted to glucose, the main substance that is used for energy production. All the excess carbohydrates are turned into fat when they aren't used as energy.

Now, what you need to remember is that you need to consume 'real carbohydrates' by choosing foods that are not processed. Replace the processed carbohydrates with natural ones like vegetables and fruits in every meal. Momentarily avoid other carbohydrates like chips, breads, pasta, fast food meals and others.

2. Have you heard of high-biological proteins? Choose them among others.

High-biological proteins are what you can think of as complete proteins. They are called such because they contain complete amino acids to provide efficient functions in terms of repairing body tissues and supplying proteins to every muscle in your body. Amino acids work like a team: when one is missing, they cannot function well. So it is good to invest in high-biological proteins by eating natural and grass-fed meats and produce. This includes turkey, beef, chicken, lamb, pork and other animal proteins.

3. There are healthy fats, of course.

If you think that fats are the only culprits of weight gain, you are definitely wrong. Your body also needs fats in order to function well as these substances contribute to temperature control, metabolism regulation and lubrication of vein and arteries. So, have a moderate intake of healthy fats, including avocadoes, coconut oil, olive oil, nuts, olives, seeds and butter. Just remember to consume about 2-3 teaspoons of these fats at every meal.

These are the three easy steps that you can always remember for you to have a significant weight loss. Start on these rules and you are off to a good start. It is good to remember that metabolism is as complex as our brain, so the notion of calorie counting does not really apply to all.

The basis of a healthy weight should come from consuming the right amount and kinds of food or to simply put it: the right balance of food. So start your meal right today by investing more on real carbohydrates, high-biological proteins and healthy fats.

The Essence of Protein to Muscles

Proteins are essential to help tissues repair themselves and supply a leaner body structure. There are so many uses of proteins you may never know. In fact, they can also be used as energy when the carbohydrate sources are empty.

Aside from that, they strengthen your immune system and give you skin that is smooth in texture. It has anti-aging benefits, enhances memory and so much more. This is why proteins are pretty valuable and should be saved for their functions instead of using them as energy.

The Right Kind of Proteins

Choosing the right kind of protein is essential to give you the advantage of having a lean body mass without the risk of sore muscles. The advice below is from an expert trainer, Taoist master Tommy Kirchhoff. He studied the popular martial arts Sheng Long Fu and is the Grandmaster of Victor Sheng Long Fu. He is a versatile fitness expert and is credited for contributing effective advice to fitness enthusiasts.

Not all have known this fact: proteins are made to function equally as compared to carbohydrates and fats.

So people are so wrong when they just invest in eating chicken alone. All proteins are a definite cure for intense training and they should be eaten in the most absorbable form.

Why?

This is because muscles need an immediate source of protein to supply their needs, especially during a heavy workout. With that, you need to opt for protein powders, as they give the quickest and most absorbable type of proteins to work and repair your body tissues.

In order to find out which powdered proteins are best for you, just visit your personal trainer or sports nutritionist. You can also visit a sports house in your area or GNC stores.

Now, if you don't just have the right budget to buy these powdered proteins, which can be expensive by the way, you can opt for egg whites. The only thing that you should remember is this: you have to eat them raw and fresh.

Yes, you can get the most amino acids in raw fresh eggs as compared to cooking them. The reason for this is because as soon as you cook the egg, the structure of its proteins changes significantly, making it less absorbable.

So manipulating an egg white, even if you shake, blend or stir them has effects that you may never know. In fact, your body may not even use the proteins completely.

Therefore, whenever you need the best proteins next to the powdered ones, get fresh eggs, separate the yolks (since they contain too much fat and cholesterol) and swallow them up.

Chapter 9- Intermittent Fasting Paired with Proper Meal Timing

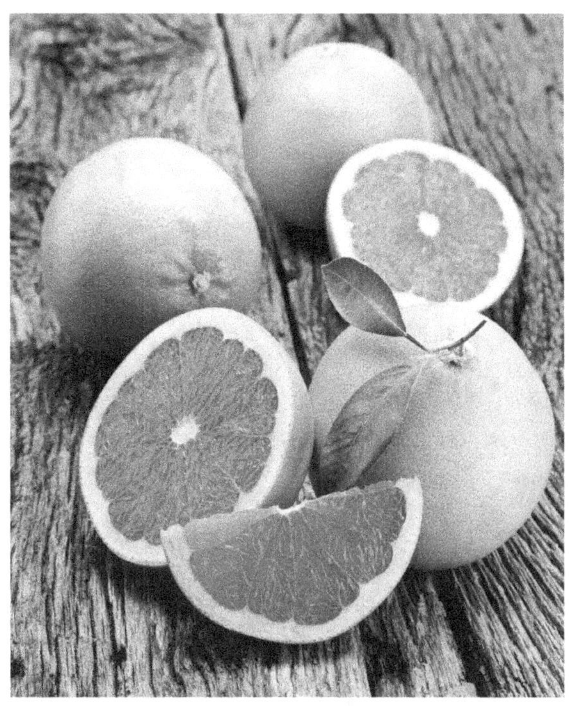

Meal timing is an essential part of a balanced diet. When we want to be on the top of our shapely figure, the right kind, amount and timing is important to balance your calories throughout the day. With that, there is no need to restrict yourself from eating lesser foods or depriving your body with the needed ingredients it should use for a day's work.

Our metabolism is different like our identity. Every individual has a different health and lifestyle profile which explains why it is hard to follow a single diet program.

A diet plan may be effective for you, but not for your friend. Even the intensity and duration of exercise may not be suitable for your friend as compared to yours. So to better understand what is actually happening inside your body, here is a basic explanation.

Breakfast Time:

Timing

• The body has fasted from sleep so there is no food intake for 8-12 hours.

• With this occurrence, the energy reserves (in the form of glycogen) are definitely low.

• This is where our muscles are in a state called mild catabolic, since the energy reserves are used for energy while there is no food intake for 8-12 hours.

• The fat stores are being used up as energy. Thus, it is being burned and mobilized.

Your metabolic goal at this time is to replenish the glycogen stores that were used from the fasting hours. You also need to stop your muscles from catabolism so that you will not acquire a state of muscle wasting. Along with that, you also need to support the continuous metabolism of fat.

To do that, you need to have a combination of high quality proteins that are absorbable enough to quickly replenish your muscles from fasting, like eggs and lean meats. You can also mix simple with complex carbohydrates to quickly replenish energy and at the same time, gradually release some of it as you go along your daily routine.

Fat is also important, so make sure to consume essential fatty acids. With that, you can eat walnuts, seeds and avocadoes. You can also make use of little amount of oil like canola oil or flax seed oil.

AM Snack

• The level of your glucose is already gradually balancing out

• The feeling of hunger is increased

Your metabolic goal: give your muscles the strength they need by consuming proteins and enough carbohydrates. It is good to further balance out your glucose level and at the same time, replenish protein stores.

To do that: You need to mix proteins and carbohydrates just enough to attain your metabolic goal. Consider foods with low-glycemic index and you can drink protein shakes, whey proteins from milk and fresh egg whites.

Lunch Time

• The morning snack that you have eaten is burned as energy and you may need more for a full day's work.

Your metabolic goal is to provide your muscles with sufficient calories with carbohydrates and proteins. Lunch can be your largest meal as compared to breakfast and dinner since you will work more after.

To do this, simply mix high-protein meat products like beef or chicken, then opt for high-fiber and low-glycemic carbohydrates. It is also good to invest in essential fatty acids.

PM Snack

• The levels of the glucose in your body are now deteriorating.

• With a few hours of mild fasting, your muscle is in a metabolic state again.

At this time, your metabolic goal is to gradually level your glucose up and stop the muscles from being catabolized.

To do this: Simply choose a snack that is enough to keep you replenished until dinner. Eat proteins that are slowly absorbed like cooked eggs. As for the carbohydrates, choose the ones that are low in sugar but are dense in calories.

Dinner Time

• Your muscles are anabolic as they prepare for another 8-12 hours of fasting during a sleep. This is up until about 12 in the morning.

Your metabolic goals should support your muscles while they are in an anabolic stage so the catabolic state will not impose any health problems in the long run.

With that, you need to eat types of foods that are low in calories but rich in protein. Choose proteins that are slowly absorbed like beef, pork and chicken. Invest in high-fiber carbohydrates and essential fatty acids.

Calorie Deficit, a New and More Effective Approach

Fortunately, some weight loss advocates are trying to shift approaches, from low-calorie diets to less stressful methods. And they base the shift on something that's simple and logical – calorie deficit.

When you are overweight, it only means one thing; you have fat deposits in your body that your metabolism can't process. The question is why your metabolism can't do that. The answer is you are taking more calories than your metabolism can handle. Does this mean that you have to starve yourself in order to lose weight? Of course not, you will be risking your health if you do that and you will end up dealing with worse problems than before.

The key to losing weight without experiencing a whole range of issues is to create a calorie deficit, which simply means that you eat fewer calories than your body demands. Fewer calories are the keywords, not zero-calories.

When you take in fewer calories and you work out, your body starts burning your fat deposits to supply you with the energy you need for the workouts. Naturally when your body burns fat deposits every day you will not be far away from your ideal weight.

Advantages

The calorie deficit approach has many advantages that are not present in drastically reduced weight loss diets. You do not need specially prepared meals to ensure the required calorie intake levels. All you need to is to eliminate some of the calorie loaded foods you are in the habit of eating. Your body won't be deprived of energy which allows it to function normally and you will feel good as you lose weight.

Aside from reducing the calories, your diet has to be as nutritionally balanced as you can make it. You want the natural body cleansers in it to help your metabolism work more efficiently.

You need the proteins and other nutrients that promote good health.

Benefits

One of the benefits of the calorie deficit approach to losing weight is your health is never compromised; instead, you can become healthier. And unlike low calorie diets that make it difficult for you to protect gains because the deprivation will make the foods you used to eat hard to resist, with this approach since its slower the diet will be a habit by the time you have realized your weight reduction goals.

Chapter 10- More Reasons to Love Intermittent Fasting

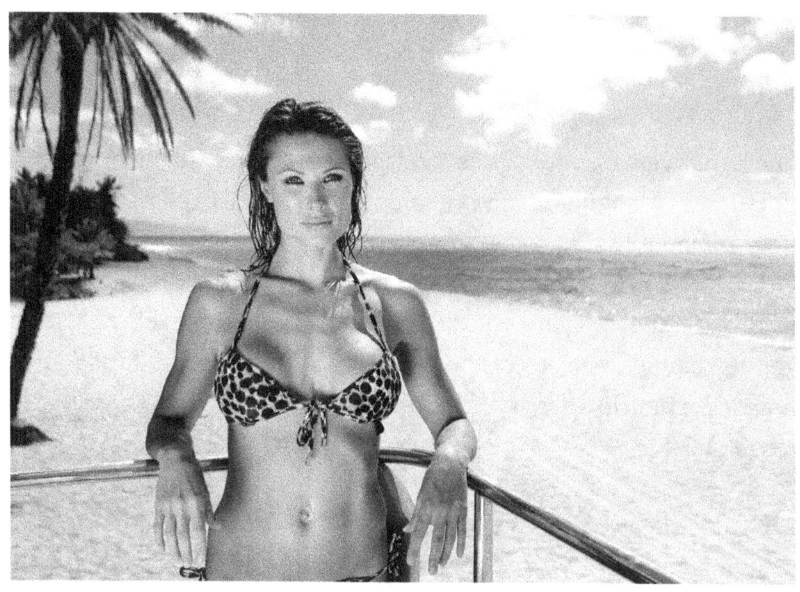

Each one of the following foods is clinically proven to promote weight loss. These foods go a step beyond simply adding no fat to your system – they possess special properties that add zip to your system and help your body melt away unhealthy pounds. These incredible foods can suppress your appetite for junk food and keep your body running smoothly with clean fuel and efficient energy.

You can include these foods in any sensible weight-loss plan. They give your body the extra metabolic kick that it needs to shave off weight quickly.

A sensible weight loss plan calls for no fewer than 1,200 calories per day. But Dr. Charles Klein recommends consuming more than that, if you can believe it – 1,500 to 1,800 calories per day. He says you will still lose weight quite effectively at that intake level without endangering your health.

Hunger is satisfied more completely by filling the stomach. Ounce for ounce, the foods listed below accomplish that better than any others. At the same time, they're rich in nutrients and possess special fat-melting talents.

Apples

These marvels of nature deserve their reputation for keeping the doctor away when you eat one a day. And now, it seems, they can help you melt the fat away, too.

First of all, they elevate your blood glucose (sugar) levels in a safe, gentle manner and keep them up longer than most foods. The practical effect of this is to leave you feeling satisfied longer, say researchers.

Secondly, they're one of the richest sources of soluble fiber in the supermarket. This type of fiber prevents hunger pangs by guarding against dangerous swings or drops in your blood sugar level, says Dr. James Anderson of the University of Kentucky's School of Medicine.

An average size apple provides only 81 calories and has no sodium, saturated fat or cholesterol. You'll also get the added health benefits of lowering the level of cholesterol already in your blood as well as lowering your blood pressure.

Whole Grain Bread

You needn't dread bread. It's the butter, margarine or cream cheese you put on it that's fattening, not the bread itself. We'll say this as often as needed – fat is fattening. If you don't believe that, ponder this – a gram of carbohydrate has four calories, a gram of protein four, and a gram of fat nine. So which of these is really fattening?

Bread, a natural source of fiber and complex carbohydrates, is okay for dieting. Norwegian scientist Dr. Bjarne Jacobsen found that people who eat less than two slices of bread daily weigh about 11 pounds more that those who eat a lot of bread.

Studies at Michigan State University show some breads actually reduce the appetite.

Researchers compared white bread to dark, high-fiber bread and found that students who ate 12 slices a day of the dark, high-fiber bread felt less hunger on a daily basis and lost five pounds in two months. Others who ate white bread were hungrier, ate more fattening foods and lost no weight during this time.

So the key is eating dark, rich, high-fiber breads such as pumpernickel, whole wheat, mixed grain, oatmeal and others. The average slice of whole grain bread contains only 60 to 70 calories, is rich in complex carbohydrates – the best, steadiest fuel you can give your body – and delivers surprising amount of protein.

Coffee

Easy does it is the password here. We've all heard about potential dangers of caffeine – including anxiety and insomnia – so moderation is the key.

The caffeine in coffee can speed up the metabolism. In nutritional circles, it's known as a metabolic enhancer, according to Dr. Judith Stern of the University of California at Davis.

This makes sense, since caffeine is a stimulant. Studies show it can help you burn more calories than normal, perhaps up to 10 percent more. For safety's sake, it's best to limit your intake to a single cup in the morning and one in the afternoon. Add only skim milk to tit and try doing without sugar – many people learn to love it that way.

Grapefruit

There's good reason for this traditional diet food to be a regular part of your diet. It helps dissolve fat and cholesterol, according to Dr. James Cerd of the University of Florida. An average sized grapefruit has 74 calories, delivers a whopping 15 grams of pectin (the special fiber linked to lowering cholesterol and fat), is high in vitamin C and potassium and is free of fat and sodium.

It's rich in natural galacturonic acid, which adds to its potency as a fat and cholesterol fighter. The additional benefit here is assistance in the battle against atherosclerosis (hardening of the arteries) and the development of heart disease. Try sprinkling it with cinnamon rather than sugar to take away some of the tart taste.

Mustard

Try the hot, spicy kind you find in Asian import stores, specialty shops and exotic groceries. Dr. Jaya Henry of Oxford Polytechnic Institute in England, found that the amount of hot mustard normally called for in Mexican, Indian and Asian recipes, about one teaspoon, temporarily speeds up the metabolism, just as caffeine and the drug ephedrine do.

"But mustard is natural and totally safe," Henry says. "It can be used every day, and it really works. I was shocked to discover it can speed up the metabolism by as much as 20 to 25 percent for several hours." This can result in the body burning an extra 45 calories for every 700 consumed, Dr. Henry says.

Peppers

Hot, spicy chili peppers fall into the same category as hot mustard, Henry says. He studied them under the same circumstances as the mustard and they worked just as well. A mere three grams of chili peppers were added to a meal consisting of 766 total calories. The peppers' metabolism-raising properties worked like a charm, leading to what Henry calls a diet-induced thermic effect. It doesn't take much to create the effect. Most salsa recipes call for four to eight chilies – that's not a lot.

Peppers are astonishingly rich in vitamins A and C, abundant in calcium, phosphorus, iron and magnesium, high in fiber, free of fat, low in sodium and have just 24 calories per cup.

Potatoes

We've got to be kidding, right? Wrong. Potatoes have developed the same "fattening" rap as bread, and it's unfair. Dr. John McDougal, director of the nutritional medicine clinic at St. Helena Hospital in Deer Park, California, says, "An excellent food with which to achieve rapid weight loss is the potato, at 0.6 calories per gram or about 85 calories per potato." A great source of fiber and potassium, they lower cholesterol and protect against strokes and heart disease.

Preparation and toppings are crucial. Steer clear of butter, milk and sour cream, or you'll blow it. Opt for yogurt instead.

Rice

An entire weight-loss plan, simple called the Rice Diet, was developed by Dr. William Kempner at Duke University in Durham, North Carolina. The diet, dating to the 1930's, makes rice the staple of your food intake. Later on, you gradually mix in various fruits and vegetables.

It produces stunning weight loss and medical results. The diet has been shown to reverse and cure kidney ailments and high blood pressure.

A cup of cooked rice (150 grams) contains about 178 calories – approximately one-third the number of calories found in an equivalent amount of beef or cheese. And remember, whole grain rice is much better for you than white rice.

Soups

Soup is good for you! Maybe not the canned varieties from the store – but old-fashioned, homemade soup promotes weight loss. A study by Dr. John Foreyt of Baylor College of Medicine in Houston, Texas, found that dieters who ate a bowl of soup before lunch and dinner lost more weight than dieters who didn't. In fact, the more soup they ate, the more weight they lost. And soup eaters tend to keep the weight off longer.

Naturally, the type of soup you eat makes a difference. Cream soups or those made of beef or pork are not your best bets. But here's a great recipe:

Slice three large onions, three carrots, four stalks of celery, one zucchini and one yellow squash. Place in a kettle. Add three cans crushed tomatoes, two packets low-sodium chicken bouillon, three cans water and one cup white wine (optional). Add tarragon, basil, oregano, and thyme and garlic powder. Boil, then simmer for an hour. Serves six.

Spinach

Popeye really knew what he was talking about, according to Dr. Richard Shekelle, an epidemiologist at the University of Texas. Spinach has the ability to lower cholesterol, rev up the metabolism and burn away fat. Rich in iron, beta carotene and vitamins C and E, it supplies most of the nutrients you need.

Tofu

You just can't say enough about this health food from Asia. Also called soybean curd, it's basically tasteless, so any spice or flavoring you add blends with it nicely. A 2½ " square has 86 calories and nine grams of protein. (Experts suggest an intake of about 40 grams per day.) Tofu contains calcium and iron, almost no sodium and not a bit of saturated fat. It makes your metabolism run on high and even lowers cholesterol. With different varieties available, the firmer tofus are goof for stir-frying or adding to soups and sauces while the softer ones are good for mashing, chopping and adding to salads.

Chapter 11- More Great Food Choices for your Intermittent Fasting Diet

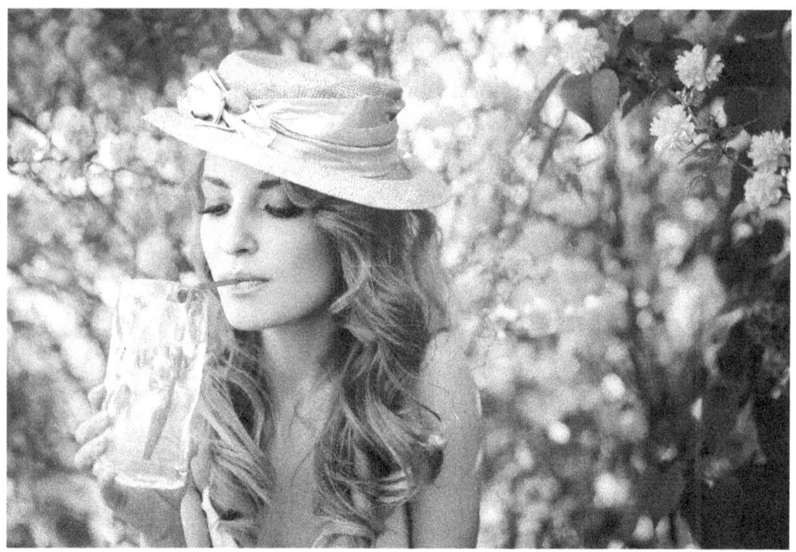

It would be unrealistic to think you could successfully lose weight and enjoy what you're eating with a mere handful of foods, no matter how delicious, nutritious and satisfying they may be. So we're going to add an extra roster of fat-fighting foods you can eat along with the great foods mentioned in the last section.

They'll lend different tastes and textures to every meal and provide a wide range of vitamins, minerals, proteins and other vital nutrients. Naturally, each one is high in fiber, low in fat and safe when it comes to sodium content, too.

Many have crunchiness and flavor we've come to desire in snack and nibbling foods. If you're like most of us, you may have a real junk food snacking habit – a habit you're going to have to change in order to slim down. Many of the foods in this section may be worthy substitutes.

Barley

This filling grain stacks up favorably to rice and potatoes. It has 170 calories per cooked cup, respectable levels of protein and fiber and relatively low fat. Roman gladiators ate this grain regularly for strength and actually complained when they had to eat meat.

Studies at the University of Wisconsin show that barley effectively lowers cholesterol by up to 15 percent and has powerful anti-cancer agents. Israeli scientists say it cures constipation better than laxatives - and that can promote weight loss, too.

Use it as a substitute for rice in salads, pilaf or stuffing, or add to soups and stews. You can also mix it with rice for an interesting texture. Ground into flour, it makes excellent breads and muffins.

Beans

Beans are one of the best sources of plant protein. Peas, beans and chickpeas are collectively known as legumes. Most common beans have 215 calories per cooked cup (lima beans go up to 260). They have the most protein with the least fat of any food, and they're high in potassium but low in sodium.

Plant protein is incomplete, which means that you need to add something to make it complete. Combine beans with a whole grain – rice, barley, wheat, corn – to provide the amino acids necessary to form a complete protein. Then you get the same top-quality protein as in meat with just a fraction of the fat.

Studies at the University of Kentucky and in the Netherlands show that eating beans regularly can lower cholesterol levels.

The most common complaint about beans is that they cause gas. Here's how to contain that problem, according to the U.S. Department of Agriculture (USDA): Before cooking, rinse the beans and remove foreign particles, put in a kettle and cover with boiling water, soak for four hours or longer, remove any beans that float to the top, then cook the beans in fresh water.

Berries

This is the perfect weight-loss food. Berries have natural fructose sugar that satisfies your longing for sweets and enough fiber so you absorb fewer calories that you eat. British researchers found that the high content of insoluble fiber in fruits, vegetables and whole grains reduces the absorption of calories from foods enough to promote width loss without hampering nutrition.

Berries are a great source of potassium that can assist you in blood pressure control. Blackberries have 74 calories per cup, blueberries 81, raspberries 60 and strawberries 45. So use your imagination and enjoy the berry of your choice.

Broccoli

Broccoli is America's favorite vegetable, according to a recent poll. No wonder. A cup of cooked broccoli has a mere 44 calories. It delivers a staggering nutritional payload and is considered the number one cancer-fighting vegetable. It has no fat, loads of fiber, cancer fighting chemicals called indoles, carotene, 21 times the RDA of vitamin C and calcium.

When you're buying broccoli, pay attention to the color. The tiny florets should be rich green and free of yellowing. Stems should be firm.

Buckwheat

It's great for pancakes, breads, cereal, and soups or alone as a grain dish commonly called kasha. It has 155 calories per cooked cup. Research at the All India Institute of Medical Sciences shows diets including buckwheat lead to excellent blood sugar regulation, resistance to diabetes and lowered cholesterol levels. You cook buckwheat the same way you would rice or barley. Bring two to three cups of water to a boil, add the grain, cover the pan, turn down the heat and simmer for 20 minutes or until the water is absorbed.

Cabbage

This Eastern Europe staple is a true wonder food. There are only 33 calories in a cup of cooked shredded cabbage, and it retains all its nutritional goodness no matter how long you cook it. Eating cabbage raw (18 calories per shredded cup), cooked, as sauerkraut (27 calories per drained cup) or coleslaw (calories depend on dressing) only once a week is enough to protect against colon cancer. And it may be a longevity-enhancing food. Surveys in the United States, Greece and Japan show that people who eat a lot of it have the least colon cancer and the lowest death rates overall.

Carrots

What list of health-promoting, fat-fighting foods would be complete without Bugs Bunny's favorite? A medium-sized carrot carries about 55 calories and is a nutritional powerhouse. The orange color comes from beta carotene, a powerful cancer-preventing nutrient (provitamin A).

Chop and toss them with pasta, grate them into rice or add them to a stir-fry. Combine them with parsnips, oranges, raisins, lemon juice, chicken, potatoes, broccoli or lamb to create flavorful dishes. Spice them with tarragon, dill, cinnamon or nutmeg. Add finely chopped carrots to soups and spaghetti sauce – they impart a natural sweetness without adding sugar.

Chicken

White meat contains 245 calories per four ounce serving and dark meat, 285. It's an excellent source of protein, iron, niacin and zinc. Skinned chicken is healthiest, but most experts recommend waiting until after cooking to remove it because the skin keeps the meat moist during cooking.

Corn

It's really a grain – not a vegetable – and is another food that's gotten a bum rap. People think it has little to offer nutritionally and that just isn't so. There are 178 calories in a cup of cooked kernels. It contains good amounts of iron, zinc and potassium, and University of Nebraska researchers say it delivers a high-quality of protein, too.

The Tarahumara Indians of Mexico eat corn, beans and hardly anything else. Virgil Brown, M.D., of Mount Sinai School of Medicine in New York, points out that high blood cholesterol and cardiovascular heart disease are almost nonexistent among them.

Cottage Cheese

As long as we're talking about losing weight and fat-fighting foods, we had to mention cottage cheese.

Low-fat (2%) cottage cheese has 205 calories per cup and is admirably low in fat, while providing respectable amounts of calcium and the B vitamin riboflavin. Season with spices such a dill, or garden fresh vegetable such a scallions and chives for extra zip.

To make it sweeter, add raisins or one of the fruit spreads with no sugar added. You can also use cottage cheese in cooking, baking, fillings and dips where you would otherwise use sour cream or cream cheese.

Figs

Fiber-rich figs are low in calories at 37 per medium (2.25" diameter) raw fig and 48 per dried fig. A recent study by the USDA demonstrated that they contribute to a feeling of fullness and prevent overeating. Subjects actually complained of being asked to eat too much food when fed a diet containing more figs than a similar diet with an identical number of calories.

Serve them with other fruits and cheeses. Or poach them in fruit juice and serve them warm or cold. You can stuff them with mild white cheese or puree them to use as a filling for cookies and low-calorie pastries.

Fish

The health benefits of fish are greater than experts imagined – and they've always considered it a health food.

The calorie count in the average four-ounce serving of a deep-sea fish runs from a low of 90 calories in abalone to a high of 236 in herring. Water-packed tuna, for example, has 154 calories. It's hard to gain weight eating seafood.

As far back as 1985, articles in the New England Journal of Medicine showed a clear link between eating fish regularly and lower rates of heart disease. The reason is that oils in fish thin the blood, reduce blood pressure and lower cholesterol.

Dr. Joel Kremer, at Albany Medical College in New York, discovered that daily supplements of fish oil brought dramatic relief to the inflammation and stiff joints of rheumatoid arthritis.

Greens

We're talking collard, chicory, beet, kale, mustard, Swiss chard and turnip greens. They all belong to the same family as spinach, and that's one of the super-stars. No matter how hard you try, you can't load a cup of plain cooked greens with any more than 50 calories.

They're full of fiber, loaded with vitamins A and C, and free of fat. You can use them in salads, soups, casseroles or any dish where you would normally use spinach.

Kiwi

This New Zealand native is a sweet treat at only 46 calories per fruit. Chinese public health officials praise the tasty fruit for its high vitamin C content and potassium. It stores easily in the refrigerator for up to a month. Most people like it peeled, but the fuzzy skin is also edible.

Leeks

These members of the onion family look like giant scallions, and are every bit as healthful and flavorful as their better-known cousins. They come as close to calorie-free as it gets at a mere 32 calories per cooked cup.

You can poach or broil halved leeks and then marinate them in vinaigrette or season with Romano cheese, fine mustard or herbs. They also make a good soup.

Lettuce

People think lettuce is nutritionally worthless, but nothing could be farther from the truth. You can't leave it out of your weight-loss plans, not at 10 calories per cup of raw romaine. It provides a lot of filling bulk for so few calories. And it's full of vitamin C, too. Go beyond iceberg lettuce with Boston, bibb and cos varieties or try watercress, arugula, radicchio, dandelion greens, purslane and even parsley to liven up your salads.

Melons

Now, here's great taste and great nutrition in a low-calorie package! One cup of cantaloupe balls has 62 calories, on cup of casaba balls has 44 calories, one cup of honeydew balls has 62 calories and one cup of watermelon balls has 49 calories.

They have some of the highest fiber content of any food and are delicious. Throw in handsome quantities of vitamins A and C plus a whopping 547 mgs of potassium in that cup of cantaloupe, and you have a fat-burning health food beyond compare.

Oats

A cup of oatmeal or oat bran has only 110 calories. And oats help you lose weight. Subjects in Dr. James Anderson's landmark 12-year study at the University of Kentucky lost three pounds in two months simply by adding 100 grams (3.5 ounces) of oat bran to their daily food intake and nothing else. Just don't expect oats alone to perform miracles – you have to eat a balanced diet for total health.

Onions

Flavorful, aromatic, inexpensive and low in calories, onions deserve a regular place in your diet. One cup of chopped raw onions has only 60 calories, and one raw medium onion (2.15" diameter) has just 42.

They control cholesterol, thin the blood, protect against cholesterol and may have some value in counteracting allergic reactions. Most of all, onions taste good and they're good for you.

Partially boil, peel and bake, basting with olive oil and lemon juice. Or sauté them in white wine and basil, then spread over pizza. Or roast them in sherry and serve over paste.

Pasta

The Italians had it right all along. A cup of cooked paste (without a heavy sauce) has only 155 calories and fits the description of a perfect starch-centered staple. Analysis at the American Institute of Baking shows pasta is rich in six minerals, including manganese, iron, phosphorus, copper, magnesium and zinc. Also be sure to consider whole wheat pastas, which are even healthier.

Sweet Potatoes

You can make a meal out of them and not worry about gaining a pound – and you sure won't walk away from the table feeling hungry. Each sweet potato has about 103 calories. Their creamy orange flesh is one of the best sources of vitamin A you can consume.

You can bake, steam or microwave them. Or add them to casseroles, soups and many other dishes. Flavor with lemon juice or vegetable broth instead of butter.

Tomatoes

A medium tomato (2.5" diameter) has only about 25 calories. These garden delights are low in fat and sodium, high in potassium and rich in fiber.

A survey at Harvard Medical School found that the chances of dying of cancer are lowest among people who eat tomatoes (or strawberries) every week.

And don't overlook canned crushed, peeled, whole or stewed tomatoes. They make sauces, casseroles and soups taste great while retaining their nutritional goodness and low-calorie status. Even plain old spaghetti sauce is a fat-burning bargain when served over pasta, so think about introducing tomatoes into your diet

Turkey

Give thanks to those pilgrims for starting the wonderful tradition of Thanksgiving turkey. It just so happens that this health food disguised as meat is good year-round for weight control.

A four-ounce serving of roasted white meat turkey has 177 calories and dark meat has 211.

Sadly, many folks are still unaware of the versatility and flavor of ground turkey. Anything hamburger can do, ground turkey can do at least as well, from conventional burgers to spaghetti sauce to meat loaf.

Some ground turkey contains skin which slightly increases the fat content. If you want to keep it really lean, opt for ground breast meat. But since this has no added fat, you'll need to add filler to make burgers or meat loaf hold together.

Four ounces of ground turkey has approximately 170 calories and nine grams of fat — about what you'd find in 2.5 teaspoons of butter or margarine. Incredibly, the same amount of regular ground beef (21% fat) has 298 calories and 23 grams of fat.

Buying turkey has become easy. It's no longer necessary to buy a whole bird unless you want to. Ground turkey is available fresh or frozen, as are individual parts of the bird, including drumsticks, thighs, breasts and cutlets.

Yogurt

The non-fat variety of plain yogurt has 120 calories per cup and low-fat, 144. It delivers a lot of protein and , like any dairy food, is rich in calcium and contains zinc and riboflavin.

Yogurt is handy as a breakfast food — cut a banana into it and add the cereal of your choice.

You can find ways to use it in other types of cooking, to — sauces, soups, dips, toppings, stuffings and spreads. Many kitchen gadget departments even sell a simple funnel for making yogurt cheese.

Yogurt can replace heavy creams and whole milk in a wide range of dishes, saving scads of fat and calories.

You can substitute half or all of the higher fat ingredients. Be creative. For example, combine yogurt, garlic powder, lemon juice, and a dash of pepper and Worcestershire sauce and use it to top a baked potato instead of piling on fat-laden sour cream.

Supermarkets and health food stores sell a variety of yogurts, many with added fruit and sugar. To control calories and fat content, buy plain non-fat yogurt and add fruit yourself. Apple butter or fruit spreads with little or no added sugar are an excellent way to turn plain yogurt into a delectable sweet treat.

About the Author

Gary Hatfield is a health buff guru. He is aware of the many methods in losing weight but Gary's aim is to turn a diet program into a lifestyle. That is what this book is all about. Gary is a certified fitness instructor and a holistic instructor as well. He uses his knowledge in both fields to come up with great diet plan.

Gary lives in Ohio with his family.